THE HEART'S LABYRINTH

NAVIGATING THE COMPLEXITIES OF CARDIAC CARE

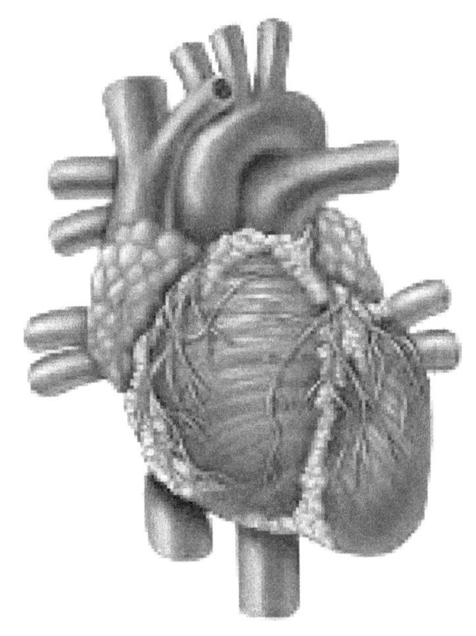

BY: DR. JADEN CLINTON

COPYRIGHT©JADENCLINTON

This book is intended for educational and informational purposes only. The content presented within is meant to contribute to the understanding and appreciation of the subject matter, health matters. Any references to specific events, names, or copyrighted material are used for the purpose of commentary, criticism, or review.

The author and publisher disclaim responsibility for any adverse effects resulting directly or indirectly from information contained in this book.

TABLE OF CONTENT

INTRODUCTION

Step into the world of " The Heart's Labyrinth: Navigating the Complexities of Cardiac Care," a profound exploration into the very core of our existence—the heart. More than a mere compilation of medical knowledge, this book shines as a beacon of hope for those grappling with the shadows of heart disease.

In the hushed confines of a hospital chamber, where the rhythmic beep of a heart monitor sets the tempo for contemplation, many have found themselves clutching the hand of a loved one, yearning for a miracle. It is from these poignant moments that the inspiration for this book arises—drawing from the stories of real-life warriors who confront heart disease with unwavering courage and resilience.

This book speaks to the daughter who takes on her first marathon in honor of her father's battle against heart disease, to the young mother who discovers strength against all odds following a heart transplant, and to the countless others who transform adversity into triumph.

Within these pages, you'll unravel the enigmatic dance of the heart, navigating the delicate balance between vulnerability and resilience. Discover how the amalgamation of modern medical advancements, lifestyle adjustments, and age-old wisdom can not only mend fractured hearts but also safeguard the life force coursing through each of us.

Here lies a testament to the indomitable human spirit's capacity for healing and a roadmap for embracing a life brimming with heartfelt vitality. Let us embark on this journey together, learning how to nurture and restore our own hearts.

This is an invitation to embrace the power within us to heal and thrive, pulsating with the rhythm of life itself.

CHAPTER ONE

UNDERSTANDING THE HEART

1.1 ANATOMY OF THE HEART

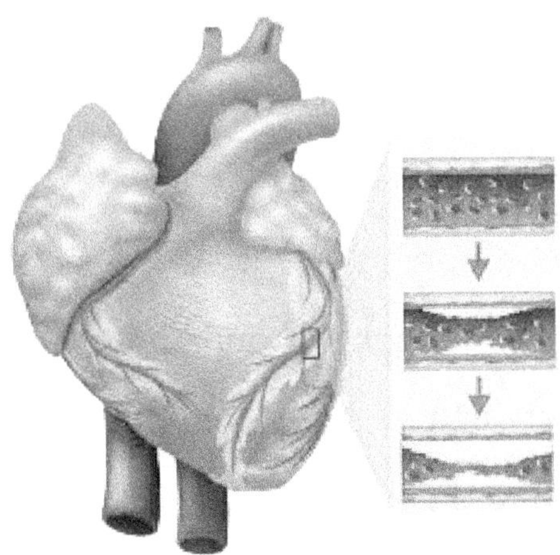

The heart, an emblem of vitality and affection, also stands as a testament to the marvels of biological craftsmanship. Join us as we embark on a journey through the intricate chambers of the heart, revealing the blueprint that propels each pulsation.

The Heart's Architectural Design

Beyond its muscular facade, the heart emerges as a multifaceted organ comprising four chambers: the dual atria and ventricles. Each chamber assumes a distinct role in the heart's perpetual mission of blood circulation. While the right-side ushers deoxygenated blood to the lungs, the left side receives oxygen-rich blood, dispatching it throughout the body's network.

Harmony of Valves

In a symphony of motion, the heart's valves perform a delicate choreography, regulating blood flow with precision. The tricuspid and mitral valves serve as sentinels between the atria and ventricles, while the pulmonary and aortic valves safeguard the heart's exits, ensuring a unidirectional flow and thwarting any backward currents.

Maestro of the Orchestra: Electrical System

Guided by its internal electrical network, the heart's rhythm unfolds like a finely orchestrated performance. Beginning at the sinoatrial node, the heart's natural pacemaker, an electrical impulse prompts atrial contraction, propagating through the atrioventricular node and ultimately stimulating ventricular contraction. This synchronized endeavor culminates in the rhythmic lub-dub, emblematic of life's heartbeat.

Venturing deeper into the heart's anatomy, we'll unravel the protective layers enfolding and nurturing this vital organ. We'll trace the paths of the coronary arteries, the lifeblood channels that sustain it, and marvel at the connective tissues that cradle the heart, granting it the freedom to beat unfettered. Comprehending the heart's intricate anatomy serves as our gateway to honoring its complexity and resilience, paving the path for a profound exploration into preserving the vigor and fortitude of this remarkable organ.

1.2 HOW THE HEART FUNCTIONS

In the vast coherence of the human body, the heart commands the spotlight. Beyond its mere anatomical presence, it serves as the relentless powerhouse driving life's intricate circulatory ballet. Join us as we embark on a journey to unveil the heart's inner workings and its graceful choreography of function.

The Melodic Pulse

Each heartbeat echoes the heart's wondrous functionality. With every rhythmic throb, the heart contracts and releases, a harmonious rhythm propelling blood through an extensive network of vessels. This cadence, akin to the soundtrack of our existence, commences shortly after conception and persists until our final moments.

Navigating the Circulatory Path

At the heart's core lies its principal mission: to circulate blood. Depleted of oxygen, blood enters the right atrium, journeys through the right ventricle, and embarks on a rejuvenating trip to the lungs for oxygenation. Reinvigorated, it returns to the left atrium, flows into the left ventricle, and disperses throughout the body—a vital expedition completed in mere seconds, yet indispensable to life's continuum.

Adapting to Life's proportion

Responsive and attuned, the heart adjusts its tempo to meet the body's demands. Whether slumbering or sprinting, it orchestrates the perfect rhythm of blood flow. A dynamic entity, it ramps up its efforts during exertion or stress, conserving energy during periods of rest.

As we step into the heart's intricacies, we'll uncover the mechanisms governing heart rate, explore how external elements like temperature and altitude influence its performance, and marvel at its innate capacity for self-renewal. Understanding the heart's function transcends mere comprehension of medical intricacies; it's a profound acknowledgment of its significance in our lives and the lives intertwined with ours.

1.3 Common Heart Conditions Explained

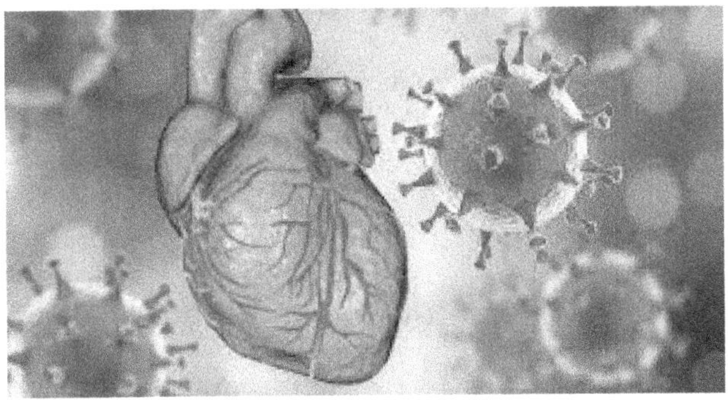

While resilient, the heart is susceptible to ailments. This chapter serves as a compassionate roadmap through the prevalent conditions that can impact this vital organ, presented with clarity and empathy.

Coronary Artery Disease (CAD)

Picture the heart's arteries as bustling highways for blood flow. When these routes are clear, traffic moves freely. However, when they become obstructed by plaque, it's akin to a gridlocked freeway, potentially leading to chest discomfort or even a heart attack. CAD stands as the foremost type of heart disease, often prompting a reevaluation of lifestyle choices.

Heart Failure

The term "heart failure" may sound ominous, but it signifies a condition where the heart's functionality diminishes, rather than ceasing entirely. It's akin to a pump operating at reduced capacity, struggling to meet the body's needs. Symptoms may include breathlessness, fatigue, and swollen extremities. Managing heart failure entails a delicate balance of medication, dietary adjustments, and physical activity

Arrhythmias

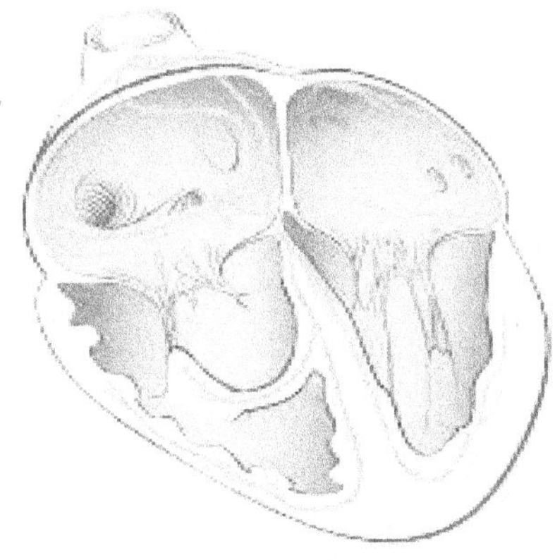

The heart's rhythm serves as its unique melody, yet occasionally, it may falter, skipping a beat or racing inexplicably. Arrhythmias manifest as irregular heartbeats, ranging from benign to potentially life-threatening variations. Understanding arrhythmias involves attuning oneself to the heart's rhythm and discerning when it deviates from its usual cadence.

Providing insights into symptoms, treatments, and the journey toward heart health, this chapter surpass mere medical discourse. It's an invitation to cultivate empathy and extend support to those grappling with these conditions on a daily basis.

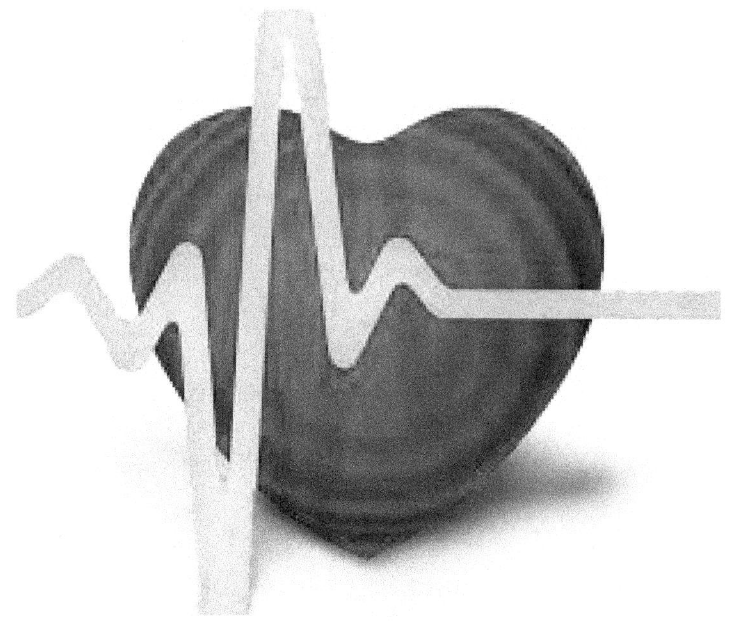

CHAPTER TWO

THE RISE OF THE HEART DISEASE

2.1 Historical Perspective on Heart Health

Venturing into a voyage through the archives of heart health unveils a narrative as ancient as humanity itself. This chapter pays homage to the trailblazers who paved the path for modern cardiology and traces the evolution of our comprehension of the heart.

Echoes of Antiquity

Ancient civilizations recognized the heart's significance, though their interpretations leaned towards symbolism rather than empirical study. Egyptians revered the heart as the seat of life and emotion, while Greek scholars like Hippocrates and Galen initiated early explorations into its function and structure, albeit through lenses that now seem archaic.

The Renaissance Resurgence

The Renaissance sparked a renaissance in anatomical inquiry, leading to profound insights into the heart. Pioneering works by figures such as Andreas Vesalius and William Harvey shattered age-old misconceptions, unveiling the heart's true role in orchestrating the circulation of blood throughout the body.

The Pulse of Modernity

The 20th century heralded a seismic shift in cardiac understanding. Innovations like the electrocardiogram (EKG) and advancements in surgical techniques ushered in a new era of cardiac care. Visionaries like Helen Taussig and Charles Dotter pushed the boundaries of possibility, transforming heart disease from a grim prognosis to a manageable, and often curable, condition.

As we contemplate the historical panorama of heart health, we not only glean knowledge but also foster a deep appreciation for humanity's tireless pursuit of heart-related enlightenment and healing. This chapter serves as a tribute to that relentless pursuit, reminding us that each stride forward represented a beacon of hope, illuminating the path toward the life-preserving wisdom we cherish today.

2.2 Modern Lifestyle and Heart Disease

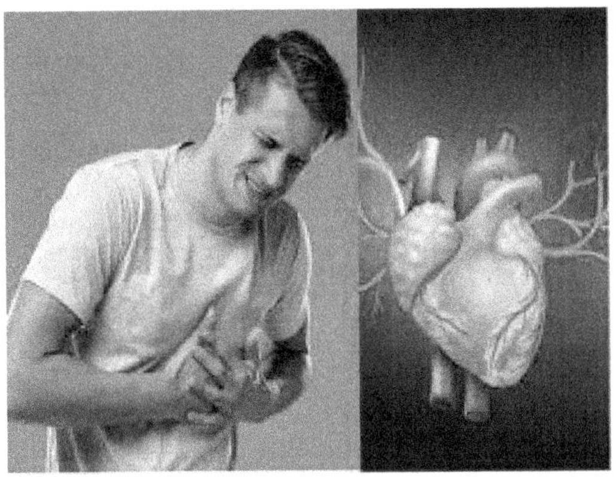

In the fabric of contemporary existence, our hearts beat to the rhythm of constant evolution. This chapter plunges into the intricate interplay between modern lifestyles and the well-being of our most vital organ.

The Velocity of Modernity

Our world races forward at an unrelenting pace, and amidst this whirlwind, stress becomes an unwelcome companion. The demands of everyday life leave scant room for reprieve, placing undue strain on the heart. We'll delve into how the incessant pressure of perpetual connectivity can elevate blood pressure and heart rate, laying the groundwork for heart-related ailments.

The Price of Convenience

Modern dietary choices epitomize convenience—fast food, processed indulgences, and sugary treats abound. While these culinary shortcuts offer time-saving benefits, they exact a heavy toll on heart health. We'll scrutinize the repercussions of diets rich in fats, salts, and sugars, unraveling their intricate links to obesity and diabetes, formidable adversaries of heart well-being.

Inactivity in an Inactive World

Our surroundings increasingly cater to sedentary habits over active lifestyles. From desk-bound occupations to binge-watching marathons, physical inertia has become the norm. This chapter sheds light on how a sedentary existence compromises heart strength and circulatory vitality, while offering strategies to counteract these deleterious effects.

Amidst the labyrinth of contemporary challenges, tales of triumph emerge—stories of individuals who've reclaimed their health by embracing heart-smart choices. This section serves not only as a cautionary narrative but also as a compass for navigating the complexities of modern living while prioritizing the well-being of our hearts.

2.3 Global Statistics and Trends

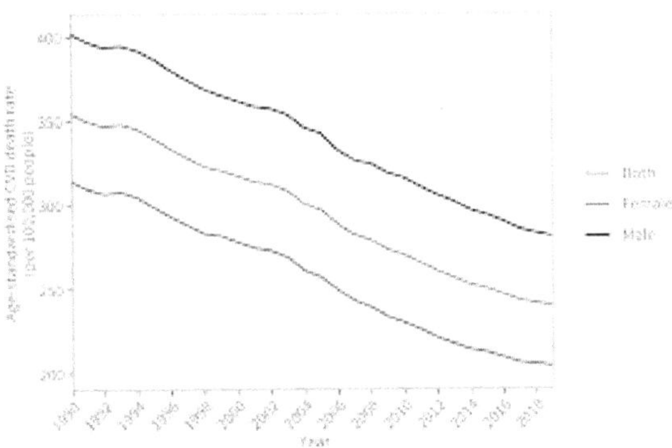

As our gaze spans the globe, the narrative of heart disease unfolds in a tapestry of numbers and trends, revealing a story of progress intertwined with challenges. This chapter offers a panoramic view of the worldwide landscape of heart health, illuminating statistics that bring clarity to the magnitude of the issue.

The Weight of Heart Disease

Heart disease remains a formidable foe, claiming millions of lives annually and retaining its status as the leading cause of death worldwide. With over half a billion individuals globally affected by cardiovascular diseases, the toll is profound, culminating in 20.5 million deaths in 2021 alone[1]. These figures, representing nearly a third of global mortality, underscore the pervasive threat posed by heart disease.

Prevention: A Beacon of Hope

Amidst the somber statistics, a glimmer of hope emerges. Up to 80% of premature heart attacks and strokes are preventable[1]. Advances in medical science and heightened awareness have armed us with the means to combat this silent assailant. However, disparities in access to life-saving interventions persist, disproportionately burdening low- and middle-income nations[1].

A Dichotomy of Realities

The battle against heart disease is characterized by stark contrasts. While affluent nations have witnessed a decline in cardiovascular fatalities owing to robust healthcare infrastructures and proactive policies, progress has stagnated or regressed in other regions[1]. Sub-Saharan Africa, for instance, grapples with elevated blood pressure levels and environmental pollutants, confronting unique obstacles in tackling heart disease[2].

Forging Ahead

Looking towards the purview, the global trajectory of heart disease mandates a unified endeavor to bridge the chasm between awareness and action. While the world possesses the knowledge to mitigate cardiovascular risks, it is imperative that this knowledge transcends borders and reaches every corner of the globe. This chapter transcends mere data; it serves as a clarion call to elevate heart health to a universal imperative.

In the ensuing pages, we go deeper into these statistics and trends, providing an expansive overview of the state of heart health worldwide. It's not just a snapshot of our current position but a roadmap guiding us towards a future where heart health knows no boundaries.

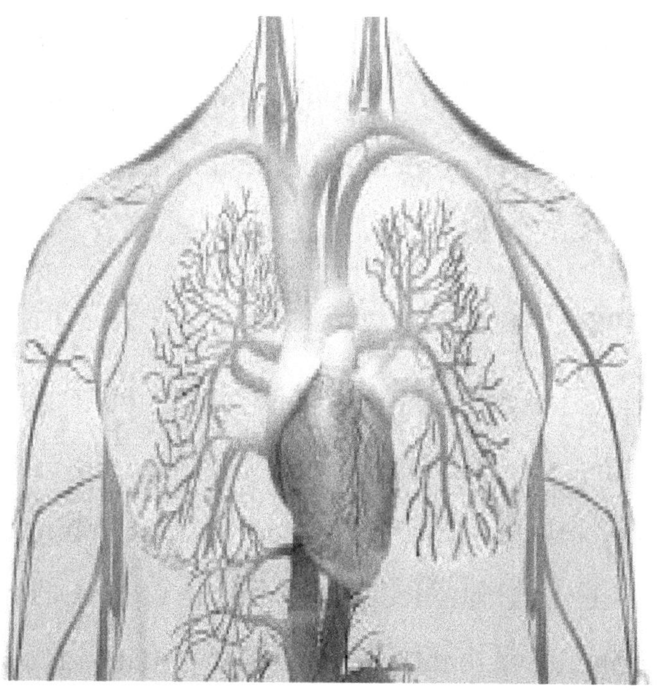

CHAPTER THREE

Risk Factors for Heart Disease

3.1 Genetic Predispositions

Within the intricate strands of our DNA lies the essence of our being—a legacy woven across generations. In this chapter, we embark on a journey through the genetic landscape that predisposes some to heart disease, exploring the nuanced interplay between inheritance and well-being.

Tracing Heart Health in the Family Tree

Much like inheriting physical traits, our genetic heritage can also shape our susceptibility to heart disease. Specific genes may elevate the risk of conditions such as high cholesterol or hypertension. Through tales of families confronting this genetic legacy, we delve into how they navigate these inherent risks together.

Navigating Your Genetic Landscape

Understanding your familial medical history serves as a compass for potential health challenges. It's not about foreseeing fate but rather about empowerment through knowledge and proactive measures. We'll unravel how genetic counseling and testing offer insights into heart health and discuss actionable steps for those at heightened genetic risk.

Genetic Influence: Not a Sole Decider

While genetics exert influence, they do not dictate our health trajectory entirely. Lifestyle choices and environmental factors wield considerable sway over how our genetic predispositions manifest. Empowered by understanding, this chapter equips you with strategies to mitigate genetic vulnerabilities, emphasizing that with informed decisions, you can chart your heart's course.

As we navigate the network of genetics, our focus remains on human stories, highlighting real-world implications and the individual's agency in shaping health outcomes.

This chapter serves as a passage of revelation, enlightenment, and optimism, reminding us that while genes may sculpt us, they do not define us.

3.2 Environmental and Lifestyle Risks

In the intricate fabric of existence, our surroundings and daily choices wield profound influence over the health of our hearts. This section unfolds a narrative surrounding external factors that can sway the balance toward heart disease, interwoven with the everyday decisions that sculpt our heart's trajectory.

Breathing in the Atmosphere

Our hearts are intimately entwined with the world we inhabit, and the quality of the air we breathe holds significance. Pollution, with its clandestine particles, can instigate inflammation within the heart's arteries, amplifying the risk of heart attacks and strokes. Through exploration, we'll uncover the ramifications of environmental pollutants on heart health and spotlight communities uniting to purify the air in the name of heart well-being.

Navigating the Tides of Stress

Stress emerges as an unseen tempest, casting a shadow over our cardiovascular health. Prolonged stress can elevate blood pressure, a precursor to heart disease. Within this segment, we'll delve into the science underpinning stress and its impact on the heart, alongside introductions to individuals who've pioneered innovative stress-management techniques to safeguard their heart health.

Lifestyle Choices: A Balancing Act

Each day presents choices that reverberate through our heart's vitality, from dietary preferences to sleep habits. Sedentary lifestyles, unhealthy diets, and tobacco consumption stand as stark examples of choices that imperil our hearts. Yet amidst the risks, there exists a beacon of hope—this chapter not only delineates potential hazards but also celebrates the transformative potential of positive change, offering practical guidance and uplifting anecdotes of triumph.

As we cover the field of environmental and lifestyle influences on heart disease, our narrative remains tethered to the personal and relatable. This chapter transcends a mere enumeration of risks; it fosters a dialogue on existence, our interconnected world, and the harmonious coexistence we can forge with our hearts.

3.3 The Impact of Stress and Emotions

Beyond its biological functions, the heart serves as a repository of our emotions and stress. This chapter delves into the intricate interplay between our emotional states and stress levels, shedding light on a deeply human aspect of heart health that resonates universally.

Emotions: The Heart's Symphony

Our hearts dance to the rhythm of our emotions—joy ignites a flutter, while sorrow weighs it down. We'll unravel the physiological responses of the heart to our emotional landscapes, examining how chronic negative emotions, like anger and sadness, can impact heart health. Through personal narratives, we'll witness how emotions not only stir within the heart but also leave an indelible mark on its well-being.

Stress: A Quiet Aggressor

Stress emerges as an invisible adversary, silently taxing the heart over time. It triggers the 'fight or flight' response, unleashing hormones that momentarily escalate heart rate and blood pressure. However, chronic stress resembles a perpetually revved engine, gradually eroding the heart's resilience. Amidst discussion on stress management strategies, we'll interlace real-life tales of individuals who've triumphed over stress, safeguarding their heart's vitality.

Nurturing the Heart through Positivity

Just as negative emotions can harm, positive emotions possess healing potential. Happiness, love, and laughter act as salves, enhancing blood vessel function and mitigating stress hormones. This section will spotlight the science underlying the cardiovascular benefits of positive emotions, alongside uplifting anecdotes of individuals harnessing this power to fortify their heart health.

Within this chapter unfolds a narrative that cross the heart with our innermost sentiments, underscoring the significance of tending to our emotional well-being alongside our physical health. It serves as a poignant reminder that the heart not only feels but also responds, heals, and thrives—in a tangible, physiological manifestation of our emotions.

CHAPTER FOUR

Symptoms and Early Detection

4.1 Recognizing the Warning Signs

Within the involute dialogue of the body, the heart communicates through subtle whispers and occasional alarms—a language that requires attentive listening. This chapter is a roadmap for deciphering these signals, empowering you to heed your body's cues before they crescendo into urgent pleas for assistance.

Chest Discomfort: The Telltale Sign

Chest pain or discomfort, often likened to squeezing, pressure, or fullness, serves as the quintessential symptom of underlying heart issues. It's the body's clarion call, signaling distress within the heart's realm. Through exploration, we'll navigate the diverse manifestations of chest pain associated with heart conditions, interwoven with firsthand narratives of individuals who heeded these signals, precipitating timely intervention.

Beyond the Chest: Subtle Whispers

Heart ailments don't always announce their presence with chest pain. Sometimes, it's the subtle breathlessness during routine activities, unexplained fatigue, or even symptoms akin to indigestion. We'll explore into these understated warning signs, underscoring the significance of early detection and its transformative impact.

Listening to the Heart's Murmurs: A Women's Perspective

Women may encounter heart disease through a lens distinct from men, with symptoms that often evade easy recognition. From jaw discomfort to sudden spells of dizziness, we'll spotlight the nuanced warning signs unique to women, buoyed by firsthand accounts from those who've traversed these paths.

In this section, we won't merely enumerate warning signs; we'll equip you with the acumen to recognize and respond to them. It's a handbook for attuning yourself to your body's language and a call to action to seize control of your heart health. Remember, acknowledging these warning signs isn't about succumbing to fear; it's about embracing empowerment and summoning the fortitude to act.

4.2 The Importance of Regular Check-Ups

In life's journey, regular check-ups serve as crucial guideposts along the path to heart health. This chapter embarks on a candid discussion, illuminating why these appointments transcend mere routines, evolving into pivotal moments of care within our lives.

Fostering Preventive Care

Preventive care stands as the bedrock of well-being. Just like a finely tuned engine, our bodies thrive on regular upkeep. We'll delve into how routine heart check-ups act as sentinels, intercepting issues before they snowball into serious health concerns. Through poignant anecdotes, we'll witness the transformative impact of a routine doctor's visit on individuals' lives.

Forging Bonds with Your Cardiologist

Beyond a medical practitioner, your cardiologist becomes a trusted ally in your heart health journey. Regular check-ups cultivate a relationship grounded in an intimate understanding of your heart's journey. We'll unravel the advantages of having a healthcare partner versed in the intricacies of your heart's story, capable of tailoring care to your unique needs.

Navigating the Check-Up Terrain

What unfolds during a heart check-up? From blood pressure assessments to cholesterol screenings, we'll demystify each facet of the process, guiding you through its intricacies. You'll gain insights into the requisite tests, decipher the significance of results, and grasp how they shape your health choices.

Inside this book, we'll underscore that regular check-ups epitomize acts of self-care and self-worth. They symbolize a steadfast commitment not only to your heart but also to the vitality it sustains. By chapter's end, you'll perceive these check-ups not as burdensome chores but as indispensable components of a vibrant, healthy existence.

4.3 Advances in Diagnostic Technology

As we stand at the cusp of a new medical epoch, cardiology undergoes a paradigm shift propelled by technological marvels that redefine how we detect heart disease. This chapter peers into the future, where state-of-the-art tools and methodologies infuse fresh optimism into the hearts of those vulnerable to cardiac conditions.

Embarking on the Digital Journey

In this era of digitization, our comprehension of the heart grows sharper and more personalized. Wearable sensors and adaptable electronics now offer continuous monitoring of cardiac health, furnishing a torrent of data once deemed unfathomable. These devices morph from passive observers to proactive custodians, sounding alerts at the faintest hint of potential issues, averting crises before they burgeon.

A Glimpse through Augmented Vision

Imaging technologies, the windows into the heart's realm, undergo a renaissance of precision and insight. Novel techniques render images with unprecedented clarity, granting glimpses into the heart's structure, function, and blood flow in real-time, sans invasive procedures. These advancements unveil vistas once obscured, ushering in an era of unparalleled diagnostic precision.

Unraveling Molecular Mysteries

At the molecular frontier, diagnostic methodologies unearth the cryptic markers of heart disease. Progress in genomic analysis unveils the genetic bedrock of cardiac conditions, laying the groundwork for bespoke treatments and preventive measures. Biomarkers emerge as sentinels of early detection, affording glimpses into cardiac health through mere blood samples.

The Dawn of AI-Assisted Diagnosis

Artificial intelligence and machine learning burgeon into stalwarts of cardiovascular diagnosis. Armed with data analytics prowess, these technologies discern patterns and forecast outcomes with unprecedented accuracy. They stand as silent sentinels, augmenting physicians' diagnostic acumen, enhancing the precision and timeliness of assessments.

In this book, we'll cover these technological frontiers, knitting a narrative that intertwines human ingenuity with technological leaps. It's a testament to our strides in decoding heart disease, offering a tantalizing glimpse of the transformative journey ahead. Remember, each technological leap signifies a stride toward a future where heart disease relinquishes its grip, becoming a hurdle we surmount with resolve.

CHAPTER FIVE

Nutrition for a Healthy Heart

5.1 Heart-Healthy Diet Basics

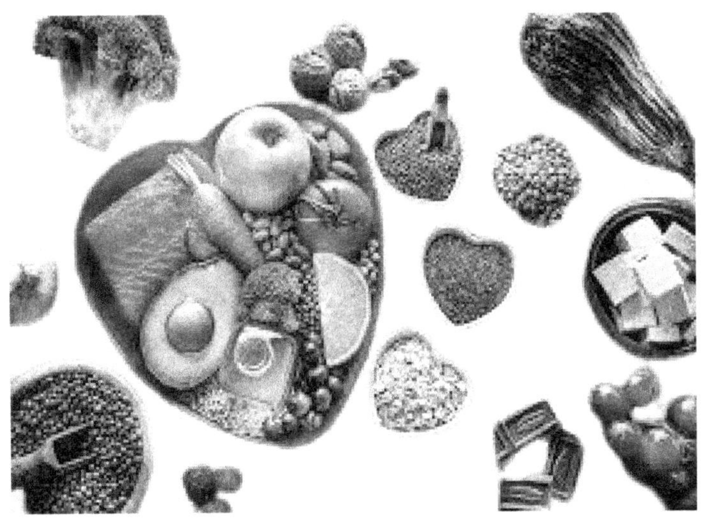

Embarking on a heart-healthy diet isn't about deprivation—it's about abundance. This chapter revels in the flavors, variety, and joy that nourishing foods bring, guiding you through the essentials of supporting your body's vital engine.

The Pillars of Heart Wellness

At the core of a heart-healthy diet lie whole grains, lean proteins, vibrant fruits and vegetables, and nourishing fats.

We'll unravel the nutritional science underpinning these choices, illustrating how each element contributes to cardiovascular vitality. From the comforting embrace of oatmeal at breakfast to the heart-boosting virtues of a handful of almonds, you'll discover the culinary keys to nurturing your heart.

Decoding Fats: Allies and Adversaries

In the element of fats, not all are created equal. While trans and saturated fats pose threats to heart health, their monounsaturated and polyunsaturated counterparts stand as protective allies. This segment demystifies the fat landscape, empowering you to make informed choices that fortify your heart's resilience.

Tackling Salt and Sugar: Stealthy Enemies

Excessive salt and sugar lurk as silent adversaries to heart well-being. We'll delve into their insidious effects, elucidating how they elevate blood pressure and imperil heart health. Armed with practical strategies, you'll navigate ways to dial back their presence in your meals without compromising on flavor.

Savoring the Pleasures of Eating

This chapter isn't a rulebook—it's an ode to relishing food while nurturing your heart. You'll encounter tantalizing, heart-healthy recipes, savvy dining-out tips, and insights on transforming your kitchen into a sanctuary for heart-centered cooking.

Amidst our exploration of heart-healthy eating fundamentals, we'll maintain a warm, inviting tone, spotlighting the positive transformations that accompany mindful consumption. This chapter celebrates a lifestyle where food becomes a conduit for vitality and a gesture of love to your heart. Remember, caring for your heart is a delectable journey worth savoring.

5.2 Foods to Embrace and Avoid

Embarking on a journey toward heart health means making mindful decisions about what lands on our plates. This chapter serves as a compass, guiding you to embrace foods that shower your heart with nutrients while steering clear of those better left on the store shelf.

Embrace: Allies of the Heart

A heart-healthy diet thrives on a colorful palette of fruits, vegetables, whole grains, and lean proteins. Here's to the foods that stand by your heart:

- Fruits and Vegetables: Packed with antioxidants, vitamins, and minerals, they fortify your heart against disease.

- Whole Grains: Think oats, barley, and quinoa—rich in fiber, they keep cholesterol in check and your heart in harmony.

- Lean Proteins: From omega-3 fatty acid-rich fish like salmon to plant-powered options like lentils and chickpeas, they nurture and fortify heart muscle.

Avoid: Enemies of the Heart

Just as certain foods shield your heart, others pose risks:

- Trans Fats: These heart-harmers, often lurking in processed foods, have no place in a heart-healthy diet.

- High Sodium: Too much salt can elevate blood pressure—a stealthy adversary to heart health.

- Added Sugars: Sugary indulgences can fuel weight gain and metabolic woes that strain the heart.

Finding Balance

Lives about harmony, and so is eating. Some foods, in moderation, can complement a heart-healthy diet:

- Dairy: opt for low-fat or fat-free varieties to savor calcium sans the added fat.

- Eggs: Once frowned upon, eggs have redeemed themselves. Enjoy them in moderation.

- Caffeine: A cup of joe in moderation can actually benefit heart health, but excessive intake might set your heart racing.

In this chapter, we'll step into these foods, offering savvy tips for making heart-wise choices. From delectable recipes to navigating grocery aisles and dining out, we've got you covered.

Remember, every bite is a chance to shower love on your heart. This chapter isn't about restriction—it's about empowerment and relishing the bounty of foods that can help you savor a life brimming with vitality.

5.3 Planning a Balanced Meal

Crafting a balanced meal is akin to composing a symphony—each ingredient harmonizes to create a delightful and healthful experience. This chapter serves as your maestro, guiding you through the art of orchestrating meals that resonate with nutrition and taste, all in harmony with your heart's well-being.

The Plate as Your Canvas

Visualize your plate as an artist's palette, with each segment adorned with the hues of different food groups. We'll introduce you to portion control and the delicate balance of macronutrients. Learn the art of filling your plate—half with vibrant vegetables and fruits, a quarter with nourishing whole grains, and the remainder with lean proteins. It's a visual symphony that's both pleasing to the eye and nurturing for the heart.

Timing Matters

As crucial as what you eat is when you eat it. Discover the rhythm of meals—why starting your day with a nutritious breakfast sets the tone for heart health, and how embracing smaller, frequent meals keeps your metabolism in sync.

Flavorful Enhancements

Healthy eating need not sacrifice flavor. Herbs and spices are culinary magicians, elevating dishes without relying on salt or fat. Learn how to wield these flavor enhancers to transform even the simplest meal into a heart-healthy feast.

Savoring the Moment

Eating isn't merely a physical act; it's an occasion. Mindful eating is about relishing each bite and being present in the moment. Discover how to tune into your body's hunger and fullness cues, transforming mealtime into a mindful ritual of appreciation.

In this chapter, we twist nutritional principles with the joy of eating, equipping you with the skills to craft meals that nurture both body and spirit. Remember, planning a balanced meal isn't just about following rules—it's about reveling in the culinary journey and honoring the vitality that food brings. Let's embark on this delicious adventure together, one plate at a time.

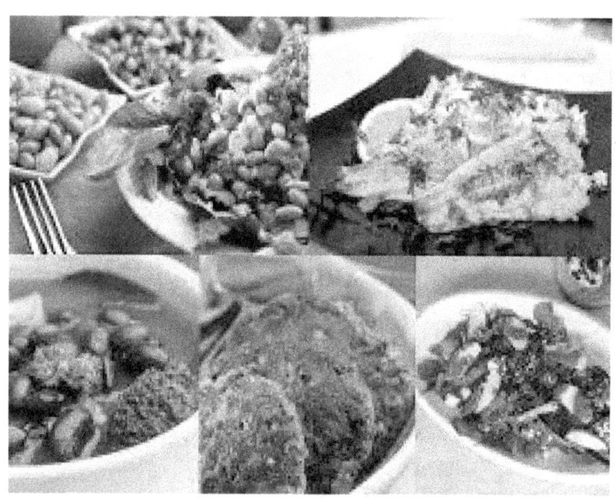

CHAPTER SIX

Exercise and Heart Health

6.1 The Role of Physical Activity

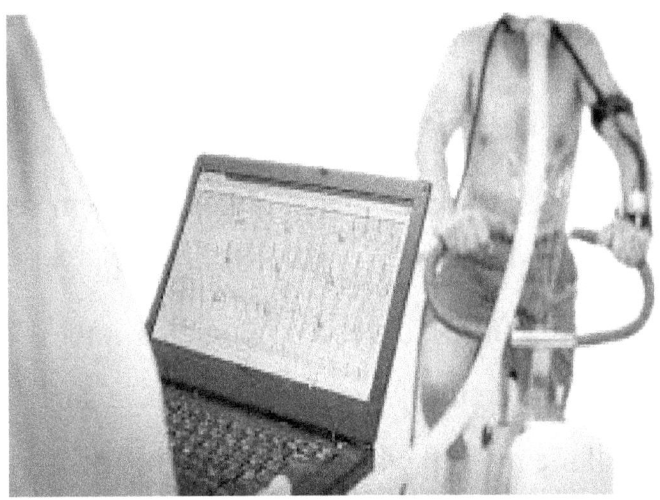

In the symphony of our well-being, physical activity serves as the rhythmic beat—it sets the tempo and mood for our heart's vitality. This chapter celebrates movement and its indispensable role in fortifying our hearts, keeping them resilient and strong.

Exercise as Therapy

Physical activity is nature's remedy for heart health. It fortifies the heart muscle, enhances blood circulation, and regulates weight and blood pressure. We'll explore how regular exercise can rival, or even surpass, medication in managing certain heart conditions. Through inspiring anecdotes, we'll witness individuals who've waltzed, strolled, and jogged their way to heart health.

Discovering Your Groove

Not everyone is destined for marathons or gym sessions, and that's perfectly fine. The key is to find an activity that brings you joy and seamlessly integrates into your life. Whether it's gardening, swimming, or a leisurely walk, we'll unveil the myriad ways to elevate your heart rate and invigorate your body.

The Science Behind Sweat

Exercise transcends calorie burn—it orchestrates biochemical shifts that benefit the heart. We'll uncover how physical activity unleashes endorphins, enhances cholesterol profiles, and dampens stress hormones, all of which contribute to a happier, healthier heart.

Fostering a Sustainable Routine

Embarking on an exercise regimen is one feat; adhering to it is another. This chapter offers pragmatic counsel on setting attainable objectives, monitoring progress, and sustaining motivation. We'll address common hurdles to exercise and impart strategies to integrate physical activity seamlessly into your daily life.

In this section, we infuse the narrative with warmth and encouragement, spotlighting the joy of movement and its profound blessings for the heart. Remember, the role of physical activity in heart health extends beyond science—it's about the experience—the breeze against your skin, the earth beneath your feet, and the surge of vitality with every stride. Let's embrace the potency of physical activity and let it guide us toward a life brimming with heart-healthy vigor.

6.2 Tailoring an Exercise Regimen

Crafting an exercise regimen is like tailoring a suit—it should fit you perfectly. This chapter is all about creating a workout routine that suits your lifestyle, preferences, and heart health objectives.

Assessing Your Starting Point

Before diving into fitness, it's crucial to evaluate your current health status. We'll stress the importance of consulting healthcare professionals to understand your heart health and any limitations you might have. This section will help you set achievable goals based on your assessment, ensuring your routine is both safe and effective.

Choosing Your Fabric: Selecting the Right Exercises

Like a tailor selecting fabric, you'll choose exercises that suit you. Whether it's the tranquility of yoga, the endurance of cycling, or the strength-building of weight training, we'll explore various activities and their cardiovascular benefits. You'll learn how to weave these exercises into a routine that's enjoyable and beneficial.

The Fitting Room: Adjusting Intensity and Duration

The intensity and duration of your workouts are vital. We'll discuss gradually increasing intensity to prevent injury and finding the optimal duration for your sessions. Personal stories will show how small adjustments can lead to significant heart health improvements.

Stitching It All Together: Creating a Cohesive Routine

A well-crafted exercise plan is consistent. This section offers strategies for incorporating exercise into your daily life, from scheduling workouts to finding workout buddies. We'll share stories of individuals who have built and maintained routines that transformed their heart health.

The Final Fit: Evaluating and Evolving Your Plan

Just like a tailored suit, your exercise plan needs adjustments over time. We'll talk about the importance of regularly evaluating your routine and making changes as necessary. Whether due to health changes, interests, or lifestyle shifts, your plan should evolve with you.

In this chapter, we'll tell a personal story, focusing on the journey toward heart health through exercise. Remember, crafting an exercise routine isn't just about physical benefits; it's about creating something that fits your life and brings joy to your heart. Let's lace up our shoes and take that first step together.

6.3 Overcoming Barriers to Exercise

The road to regular exercise isn't always smooth, but overcoming each obstacle is a victory for the heart. This chapter serves as a guide through the common hurdles we encounter on our fitness journey and offers strategies to conquer them with determination and grace.

Time: The Eternal Struggle

"I don't have time." It's a phrase we've all uttered. We'll discuss ways to carve out time for exercise, from treating workouts like non-negotiable appointments to incorporating physical activity into daily routines, such as taking walks during breaks or biking to work.

Motivation: Keeping the Fire Burning

Motivation can flicker like a candle in the wind. We'll explore methods to keep motivation alive, like setting clear, attainable goals, monitoring progress, and celebrating achievements. You'll hear stories of individuals who found their drive through group classes, personal challenges, or simply reveling in the joy of movement.

Confidence: Building from Within

Many struggles with confidence when it comes to exercise. "Am I doing it right?" "Do I fit in?" These doubts can hold us back. We'll offer advice on boosting exercise confidence, starting with simple activities and gradually mastering techniques, ensuring that every step build self-assurance.

Physical Limitations: Adapting with Grace

Physical limitations, whether from age, injury, or health conditions, can make exercise daunting. This chapter provides guidance on modifying exercises to suit your body, collaborating with healthcare providers to craft a safe routine, and finding inspiration in those who have adapted and thrived.

Environmental Barriers: Creating Your Space

Not everyone has access to a gym or safe outdoor areas for exercise. We'll explore ways to establish a conducive exercise environment at home or in the community and advocate for public spaces that promote physical activity.

Remember, each barrier to exercise is an opportunity for growth, not just physically, but also in determination and spirit. Let's turn these obstacles into stepping stones on the journey to a heart-healthy life.

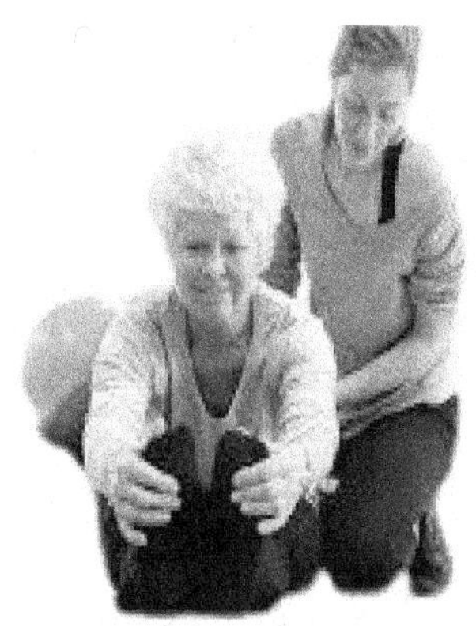

CHAPTER SEVEN

Medical Management of Heart Disease

7.1 Medications and Treatments

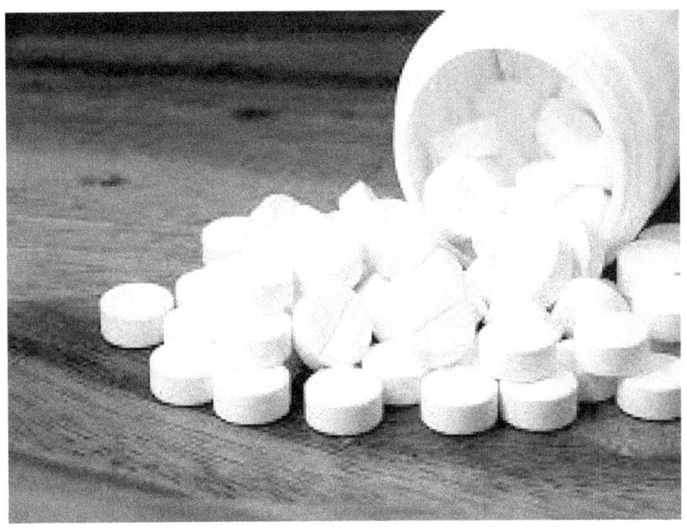

In the quest to mend broken hearts, medications and treatments stand as steadfast allies on the front lines. This chapter serves as a compassionate guide to the pharmaceuticals and procedures offering hope and healing to those grappling with heart disease.

The Medicinal Arsenal

The battle against heart disease employs a diverse array of medications, each with a specific role:

- Anticoagulants: They maintain peace, ensuring smooth blood flow without clot formation.
- Antiplatelets: These act as diplomats, preventing blood cells from sticking together and causing issues.
- Beta Blockers: Serving as shields, they safeguard the heart from stress and high blood pressure.
- ACE Inhibitors: These agents help relax blood vessels, reducing the heart's workload.

Choosing the Right Path

Selecting the appropriate treatment is a journey, involving understanding the intricacies of each medication—how they function, their advantages, and potential side effects. We'll delve into how doctors tailor treatment plans to individual needs, considering factors like age, medical history, and the specific nature of the heart condition.

Procedures and Interventions

At times, medications alone fall short, leading to medical procedures:

- Angioplasty: It's akin to clearing a traffic jam, restoring blood flow by opening up blocked arteries.
- Bypass Surgery: Think of it as constructing a detour around a closed road, establishing new pathways for blood to reach the heart muscle.

The Human Element

Behind every medication and treatment lies a team of dedicated healthcare professionals. This chapter will share narratives of the doctors, nurses, and pharmacists working tirelessly to provide care and comfort to those on the road to recovery.

A Glimpse into the Future

As we wrap up the sub chapter, we'll cast our gaze towards the horizon of heart disease treatment. The future holds promise with advances in personalized medicine, stem cell therapy, and minimally invasive procedures that could revolutionize cardiac care.

In this chapter, we'll blend informative insights with hopeful narratives, focusing on the human experiences behind the science of heart disease treatment. Remember, the journey through medications and treatments isn't solely about symptom management; it's about restoring life's rhythm and embracing the prospect of a healthier future.

7.2 Navigating Surgery Options

When the heart needs help, surgery often steps in to answer the call. This chapter is a journey through the realm of surgical options for heart disease, offering a guide to help you navigate choices that can mend the heart and restore its rhythm.

The Decision Crossroads

Choosing heart surgery is a significant decision, blending medical advice with personal considerations. It's a decision that touches both the clinical and human aspects, involving not only the patient but also their loved ones. We'll explore how to approach this choice, weighing potential benefits against risks and considering its impact on quality of life.

A Spectrum of Surgical Interventions

Heart surgery spans a spectrum of interventions, each tailored to individual needs:

- Coronary Artery Bypass Grafting (CABG): Known as bypass surgery, CABG redirects blood around blocked arteries to enhance blood flow and oxygen delivery to the heart.
- Angioplasty and Stent Placement: A less invasive option, involving inflating a balloon to widen narrowed arteries, often followed by placing a stent to keep the artery open.
- Valve Repair or Replacement: Addressing faulty heart valves, surgery can repair or replace them to ensure efficient pumping of the heart's chambers.

Preparation for the Journey

Preparing for heart surgery is itself a journey, encompassing understanding the procedure, readying the body, and establishing a support network for recovery. We'll offer a pre-surgery checklist, tips for a successful operation, and guidance on mental and emotional readiness for the path ahead.

Technological Advancements

In the operating room, technology serves as a vital ally. From robotic assistance to advanced imaging, innovations enhance the safety and effectiveness of heart surgery. We'll explore the latest advancements, including minimally invasive techniques that shorten recovery times and enhance outcomes.

The Road to Recovery

Recovery from heart surgery is as crucial as the surgery itself. It's a journey marked by patience, determination, and gradual progress. We'll outline what to expect during recovery, including potential challenges and strategies for overcoming them. Rehabilitation programs, lifestyle adjustments, and support networks all play pivotal roles in regaining strength and resuming daily activities.

Navigating Together

No one should navigate surgery alone. This chapter underscores the importance of a supportive team— comprising medical professionals, loved ones, and support groups—to accompany and assist you every step of the way. We'll share insights and encouragement from those who've traversed this path before.

Looking Ahead

As we conclude, we'll cast our gaze toward the future of heart surgery. With promising advancements in techniques and therapies, the future holds potential for less invasive, more precise, and even more successful surgeries.

In this chapter, we'll blend informative guidance with empathetic support, spotlighting the human side of heart surgery options. Remember, this ride isn't just about the heart—it's about the whole person. It's about making informed decisions that pave the way for a healthier, more vibrant life. Let's step on this journey together, with courage and optimism for what lies ahead.

7.3 The Future of Heart Disease Treatment

As we gaze towards the horizon of medical progress, the future of heart disease treatment holds the promise of innovation and hope. This chapter is a journey into the possibilities that await us—a narrative woven with the threads of scientific advancement and human aspiration.

A Century of Progress

Looking back over a century of medical progress, we've witnessed a remarkable transformation in the fight against heart disease. From early rudimentary understanding to today's sophisticated interventions, each stride forward has marked a monumental leap for humanity. The American Heart Association commemorates this journey, acknowledging past achievements while casting our vision forward to the challenges and opportunities that lie ahead.

The Vanguard of Medication

The frontier of pharmaceuticals is continually expanding, with emerging medications not only offering treatment but also prevention. Injectable drugs are simplifying treatment regimens, enhancing adherence, and promising improved outcomes. Understanding the intricate links between cardiovascular health and conditions like diabetes and obesity is shedding new light, with medications originally aimed at blood sugar control now demonstrating significant benefits for the heart.

The Digital Pulse

Technology stands poised to redefine heart care. Wearable devices capable of real-time heart health monitoring, artificial intelligence predicting risks, and telemedicine extending care to remote regions represent just the tip of the iceberg. The digital heartbeat of medicine ensures that no one is beyond reach, and everyone has access to the care they require.

The Genetic Frontier

Genetics holds the key to personalized medicine. As we unravel the complexities of the genetic code, new avenues for heart disease treatment emerge. The future may hold treatments precisely tailored to an individual's genetic profile, promising levels of precision and efficacy previously unimaginable.

Regenerative Horizons

Advancements in stem cell research and regenerative medicine are opening doors to treatments capable of repairing damaged heart tissue. The vision of healing the heart from within inches closer to reality, offering the potential to revolutionize recovery from heart attacks and heart failure.

The Collaborative Effort

The future of heart disease treatment lies not solely in the hands of scientists and clinicians but also in the collective action of society. Public and private stakeholders are urged to unite in accelerating research, clinical care, and public health initiatives. The ultimate goal is a future where optimal patient care, scientific integrity, health equity, and a world free from cardiovascular diseases are not just aspirations but tangible realities.

The Human Heart

At the heart of these advancements lies not only the organ itself but the indomitable spirit of humanity. The future of heart disease treatment weaves together technology, science, and humanity—a future where the heart is not merely treated but deeply understood and cherished.

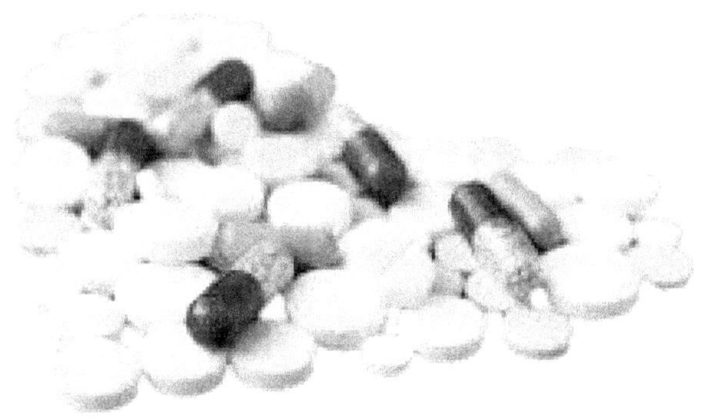

CHAPTER EIGHT

Alternative Therapies and Heart Health

8.1 Holistic Approaches to Treatment

In the realm of heart health, embracing a holistic approach to treatment is akin to composing a symphony, where each element harmonizes to create a melody of well-being. This chapter delves into the gentle yet powerful ways we can care for the heart, treating it not merely as a muscle but as an integral part of our overall well-being.

The Philosophy of Wholeness

Holistic medicine is grounded in the belief that the body, mind, and spirit are interconnected. Healing, therefore, encompasses all aspects of a person's life, seeking to restore balance and wellness on every level.

The Natural Allies

Nature provides a treasure trove of remedies to support heart health:

- **Herbs and Supplements**: From omega-3-rich fish oil to vitamin D, natural supplements can complement traditional treatments.

- **Dietary Wisdom**: A heart-healthy diet extends beyond avoidance; it's about embracing nutrient-rich foods like leafy greens, whole grains, and lean proteins.

- **The Healing Touch**: Therapies such as acupuncture and massage can enhance circulation, alleviate stress, and promote relaxation, all beneficial for the heart.

The Mind-Body Connection

Emotions deeply impact heart health; stress and anger can take a toll. Practices like meditation, yoga, and tai chi not only calm the mind but also nurture the heart, teaching us to breathe deeply, move gracefully, and live mindfully.

The Supportive Circle

Healing thrives in a supportive environment. Love and encouragement from family, friends, and support groups provide essential emotional support crucial for recovery.

Integrating Holistic Practices

Embracing holistic care doesn't mean forsaking conventional medicine; it's about integrating the best of both worlds. Collaborating with healthcare providers ensures a holistic treatment plan that addresses all aspects of heart health.

The Personal Path

Each person's journey with heart disease is unique. Crafting a personalized holistic treatment plan tailored to individual values, preferences, and needs is key.

Looking Ahead

The potential of holistic approaches in heart disease treatment is vast. With ongoing research and a deepening understanding of the heart's complexities, holistic medicine holds promise for hope and healing.

8.2 The Role of Supplements and Herbs

In the garden of heart health, supplements and herbs bloom as potential healers. This chapter takes you on a stroll through the lush fields of natural remedies, revealing their nurturing role in heart care alongside conventional treatments.

Nature's Pharmacy

Herbs and supplements have long been treasured for their healing potential, now backed by modern research. Here's a glimpse of their benefits:

- Omega-3 Fatty Acids: Derived from fish oil, these supplements are renowned for reducing triglycerides, lowering blood pressure, and mitigating arrhythmias.

- Coenzyme Q10: An antioxidant known to alleviate symptoms of congestive heart failure and aid post-heart surgery recovery.

- Red Yeast Rice: With statin-like compounds, it's considered for managing cholesterol, though caution is advised due to potential side effects.

Herbal Heartbeats

Herbs, integral to traditional medicine, are gaining recognition in cardiovascular care:

- **Hawthorn**: Esteemed for its heart-friendly traits, hawthorn may enhance coronary artery blood flow and heart muscle contraction.
- **Garlic**: Beyond seasoning, garlic exhibits potential in reducing blood pressure and cholesterol.
- **Green Tea**: Abundant in catechins, green tea may shield the cardiovascular system from oxidative stress.

The Science of Synergy

Supplements and herbs thrive when partnered with a healthy lifestyle. Diet, exercise, and stress management form the groundwork for their effectiveness.

Navigating the Natural Path

Choosing supplements and herbs demands careful attention. Quality, purity, and dosage are paramount. We'll explore how to select trustworthy brands, decipher labels, and determine suitable doses.

Interactions and Integrations

While herbs complement the body, they can interact with medications. Consulting healthcare providers, particularly for those on heart meds, is crucial to prevent adverse interactions.

The Personal Touch

Each heart health journey is unique, and so is the response to supplements and herbs. This chapter will assist in tailoring your approach to match your health needs and aspirations.

Looking Ahead

As research flourishes, the future of supplements and herbs in heart care is promising. With ongoing studies and a growing embrace of integrative medicine, their potential to bolster heart health shines brightly.

8.3 Mind-Body Techniques for Healing

In the intricate tapestry of heart health, mind-body techniques are like gentle threads weaving together the physical and the emotional. This chapter invites you into the heart's inner sanctuary, exploring practices that engage both mind and body in the quest for well-being.

The Power of Connection

Beyond its mechanical function, the heart resonates with our thoughts and feelings. The link between mind and body runs deep, influencing our heart health profoundly. From stress to joy, our mental states leave a mark on our hearts.

Healing Practices

Mind-body techniques offer a soothing remedy for life's burdens:

Meditation: A timeless practice that calms the mind and soothes the spirit. Research shows it can lower blood pressure, ease stress, and enhance blood flow to the heart.

Yoga: Beyond poses, yoga unites body and mind through breath and movement, promoting cardiovascular health and inner balance.

Tai Chi: A graceful practice that blends meditation with gentle motion, Tai Chi has been linked to reduced blood pressure and improved heart health.

The Science of Serenity

These techniques aren't just anecdotal; they're backed by science. They trigger the body's relaxation response, reducing stress, heart rate, and blood pressure. They also enhance autonomic function, regulating heart rhythm and blood pressure.

Integrating Mind-Body Practices

Incorporating these practices doesn't demand radical change. Even a few minutes of deep breathing or a weekly yoga class can make a difference. Consistency and finding what resonates with you are key.

Personal Journeys

Every heart disease journey is unique, and so is the path to healing. This chapter helps you explore mind-body practices that suit your lifestyle and preferences, offering stories of strength and inspiration along the way.

The Future of Healing

The future holds promise for mind-body techniques in heart care. With ongoing research, they may become integral to holistic heart health, nurturing not just the heart but the whole person.

CHAPTER NINE

LIVING WITH HEART DISEASE

9.1 Daily Life Adjustments

Living with heart disease isn't just about managing a condition; it's about adapting your daily routines to steer towards better health. This chapter is a roadmap for making small yet impactful changes that can transform your heart health journey.

Adjusting the Sails

Navigating life with heart disease is an art of balance. It's about tuning into your body's signals, from managing medications to planning meals and fitting in exercise. We'll delve into practical strategies to help you adjust seamlessly.

Finding Your Routine

Establishing a daily rhythm can bring stability. We'll explore crafting a schedule that prioritizes medication, exercise, and relaxation while ensuring you get adequate sleep—an often overlooked but vital aspect of heart health.

Nutrition Navigation

Nutrition is key, but it doesn't have to be complicated. We'll guide you through shopping for heart-healthy foods, deciphering nutrition labels, and preparing delicious meals. Plus, we'll tackle dining out and handling social situations with ease.

Embracing Movement

Exercise is essential for heart health, but it doesn't have to be intimidating. We'll offer tips for integrating physical activity into your day, whether it's a stroll, a swim, or a dance session. And we'll keep you motivated as you progress.

Stress Mastery

Stress is part of life, but managing it is crucial. We'll explore techniques like deep breathing and mindfulness to help you find calm amidst the chaos. You'll hear inspiring stories of others who've found peace through these practices.

Building Your Support Network

You don't have to face heart disease alone. We'll stress the importance of leaning on family, friends, or support groups for encouragement. Plus, we'll share tips for effective communication and seeking assistance when needed.

A Journey of Self-Discovery

Living with heart disease can be a path of self-exploration. It's a chance to learn more about yourself and what makes you thrive. We'll encourage you to embrace this journey, finding joy in every step forward.

Looking Forward

As we peer into the future, the landscape of heart disease management will evolve. With advancing technology and a deeper understanding of heart health, the possibilities for living well with heart disease are brighter than ever.

9.2 Emotional and Psychological Support

Living with heart disease is more than a physical journey—it deeply impacts emotional and mental well-being. From the initial diagnosis to ongoing management, individuals face a range of emotions, requiring resilience and a strong support system.

Navigating Emotional Challenges

A heart disease diagnosis can shake one's world, triggering feelings of shock, fear, and sadness. Coping with these emotions is a crucial part of the journey, as they can affect mental health and overall quality of life.

The Importance of Support

Having emotional support is vital. Whether it's from loved ones, healthcare professionals, or support groups, having a safe space to express feelings and share experiences can provide comfort and understanding.

Professional Guidance

Seeking help from therapists or counselors who specialize in chronic illness can offer valuable strategies for managing stress and improving mental well-being. Techniques like cognitive-behavioral therapy can reshape negative thought patterns and promote a positive mindset.

Building Resilience

Practices like mindfulness and relaxation techniques can foster resilience, helping individuals bounce back from adversity. Focusing on the positive aspects of life and setting achievable goals can also contribute to a more optimistic outlook.

The Heart-Mind Connection

Emotional and mental well-being directly impact heart health. Stress and negative emotions can exacerbate heart conditions, highlighting the importance of addressing emotional needs alongside physical health.

Inspiration from Others

Success stories from those who have thrived despite heart disease can provide hope and motivation. Knowing that others have overcome similar challenges can instill confidence and determination.

In conclusion, emotional and mental support are essential for navigating life with heart disease. By fostering a compassionate environment, seeking professional help when needed, and practicing resilience-building techniques, individuals can enhance their overall well-being and quality of life.

This chapter aims to shed light on the emotional and psychological aspects of living with heart disease, emphasizing the significance of holistic support in maintaining well-being.

9.3 Success Stories of Managing Heart Disease

In the **peregrinate** of battling heart disease, success stories shine as beacons of hope and resilience. These narratives are not just about survival; they are about overcoming obstacles, embracing life, and finding strength in the face of adversity. Let's delve into some inspiring tales that illuminate the path to managing heart disease with courage and determination.

Michael's Triumph over Adversity

Meet Michael, a dedicated school teacher who faced a sudden heart attack during a routine school day. Thanks to the swift action of his colleagues and medical professionals, Michael survived the ordeal. However, his journey was far from over. With a weakened heart, he embarked on a challenging road to recovery. Through disciplined lifestyle changes, including a heart-healthy diet and regular exercise, along with the unwavering support of his community, Michael not only returned to teaching but also achieved a remarkable milestone by completing his first half-marathon. His story underscores the power of positivity and the importance of a strong support system in the face of adversity.

Akila's Journey to New skyline

Then there's Akila, a young mother grappling with congenital heart disease. Traditional treatments offered limited relief until she discovered a groundbreaking minimally invasive procedure that transformed her life. With renewed vigor, Aisha became a passionate advocate for heart health, sharing her journey to inspire others facing similar challenges.

John's Technological Triumph

In the age of technology, John found innovative ways to manage his heart condition. Utilizing wearable devices to monitor his vitals and embracing telemedicine for regular consultations, John took proactive steps to safeguard his health. His story highlights the transformative impact of technology in empowering individuals to take control of their well-being.

Linda's Journey of Self-Discovery

For Linda, retirement brought a new chapter marked by heart disease. Embracing yoga and volunteering at a local heart foundation became her pillars of strength. Despite the adjustments, Linda found purpose and fulfillment in her new lifestyle, proving that life after heart disease can be meaningful and enriching.

Celebrating Collective Courage

These stories, woven together, paint a drapery of resilience and hope. They remind us of the collective strength found in sharing our journeys and supporting one another through life's challenges. Each narrative serves as a testament to the indomitable human spirit and the capacity to thrive in the face of adversity.

By sharing these inspiring accounts, this chapter aims to uplift and inspire those navigating the complexities of heart disease. It's a celebration of human triumphs, showcasing the resilience, courage, and perseverance that define the heart disease journey.

CHAPTER TEN

THE ROLE OF TECHNOLOGY IN HEART CARE

10.1 Wearable Devices and Heart Monitoring

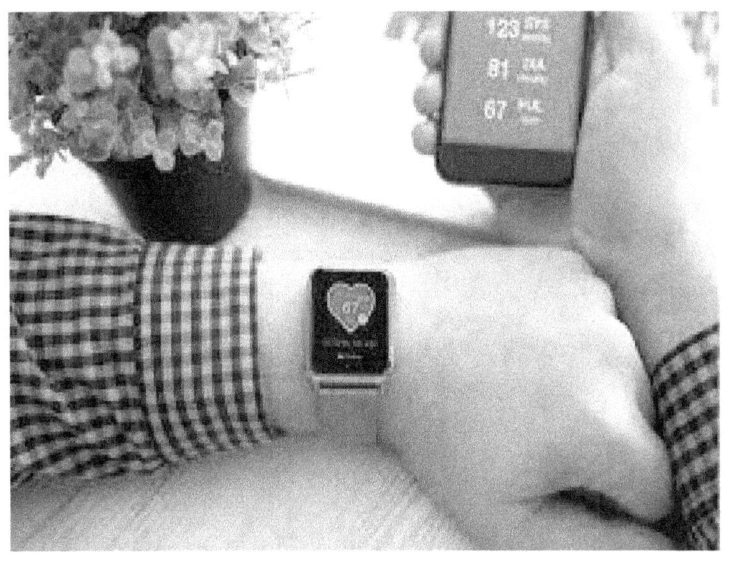

In today's digital era, technology has become an integral part of modern healthcare, especially in heart care. Wearable devices have transformed how we monitor and manage heart health, granting individuals unprecedented access to real-time data about their cardiovascular well-being.

The Evolution of Wearable Heart Monitors

While wearable heart monitors aren't new, their capabilities have evolved significantly. From basic devices measuring heart rate, we now have sophisticated gadgets tracking heart rhythm, detecting irregularities, and even predicting potential heart events.

Empowering Individuals with Data

These devices empower individuals to take an active role in their heart health. Continuous monitoring enables people to observe the immediate impact of lifestyle choices on their heart, helping them make informed decisions about daily activities and habits.

A Day in the Life with a Wearable Device

Picture starting your day with a wearable heart monitor on your wrist. It's lightweight, discreet, and constantly collecting data. It records your resting heart rate during your morning routine, notes changes as you navigate through traffic, and gently reminds you to take a brief walk at work to manage stress.

The Impact on Heart Disease Management

For those with existing heart conditions, wearable devices can be lifesaving. They serve as a safety net, alerting users to potential issues so they can seek medical attention promptly. For instance, someone with atrial fibrillation can adjust their treatment plan based on irregular heartbeat alerts.

Integration with Healthcare Systems

Data collected by these devices can be shared with healthcare providers, offering a comprehensive view of a patient's heart health over time. This integration improves communication between patients and doctors, leading to more personalized treatment strategies.

Challenges and Considerations

Despite benefits, challenges like privacy concerns and data accuracy exist. Users must understand how to interpret data and when to seek professional advice.

The Future of Wearable Heart Technology

Looking ahead, wearable heart technology holds promise. Researchers are developing devices with advanced sensors potentially detecting heart attacks in real-time, aiding emergency responders.

Wearable heart monitoring devices are more than gadgets; they enhance our understanding of heart health, bridging daily life and medical care. As technology advances, these devices will further integrate into our lives, offering a proactive approach to heart care.

This section aims to be informative yet relatable, discussing wearable devices' impact on heart health in a way resonating with human experiences. It provides readers with a thorough understanding while keeping the content engaging and accessible.

10.2 Telemedicine and Remote Care

In today's healthcare landscape, telemedicine has emerged as a game-changer, especially for patients dealing with heart disease. Telemedicine, or remote care, uses telecommunications technology to provide clinical health care from a distance, breaking down geographical barriers and granting access to medical expertise like never before.

The Rise of Telemedicine

While telemedicine isn't new, recent technological advancements have led to its widespread adoption. For heart patients, telemedicine offers a convenient alternative to traditional hospital visits, allowing for timely care without the hassle of travel.

A Peek into Telemedicine's Impact

Imagine having a video call with your cardiologist from your couch. That's the reality for many heart patients now. From routine check-ups to urgent consultations, telemedicine makes it possible. Wearable devices sync with telemedicine platforms, enabling doctors to monitor patients' heart health remotely.

Improving Patient Outcomes

Telemedicine isn't just convenient; it's effective. Studies show that remote monitoring and consultations can lead to better disease management, fewer hospital readmissions, and an overall improved quality of life. Patients feel empowered, knowing they're connected to their healthcare providers.

Bridging Gaps in Access

Telemedicine is a lifeline for those in rural or underserved areas. It brings specialized cardiac care to their doorstep, eliminating the need for long-distance travel. Expert advice, second opinions, and follow-up care are now within reach.

Navigating Challenges

While telemedicine offers many benefits, there are hurdles to overcome. Some patients may struggle with technology, and there are valid concerns about data security. Plus, nothing beats an in-person physical exam. Healthcare systems must address these issues to make telemedicine accessible to everyone.

Telemedicine in Crisis

Telemedicine truly shone during global health crises like the COVID-19 pandemic. It ensured uninterrupted care while minimizing infection risks. Heart patients, often at higher risk, could stick to their treatment plans safely.

The Bright Future Ahead

The future of telemedicine is promising, with ongoing innovations poised to enhance its capabilities. Artificial intelligence, for instance, promises more accurate diagnostics and predictive analytics. The potential for telemedicine to revolutionize heart care is vast and continually expanding.

Wrapping Up

Telemedicine isn't just a change in healthcare; it's a revolution. For heart patients, it offers security and continuity of care like never before. As technology marches forward, telemedicine will evolve, offering new and improved ways to manage heart health from a distance.

This chapter aims to make telemedicine relatable, blending technical details with real-life scenarios. It provides a comprehensive look at telemedicine's impact on heart care, presented in a way that's informative and accessible to all readers.

10.3 Innovations in Cardiac Treatment

The journey of cardiac treatment has been nothing short of remarkable, marked by constant innovation and a relentless pursuit of better outcomes for patients. Today, we find ourselves on the brink of a new era in cardiology, where groundbreaking treatments and technologies are reshaping the landscape of heart care.

Embracing Innovation in Cardiac Care

Cardiology has always been driven by a pioneering spirit. From the groundbreaking first heart transplant to the development of coronary stents, each advancement has pushed the boundaries of what's possible in treating heart disease. Now, we're witnessing the dawn of treatments once only dreamed of in science fiction.

Exploring Cutting-Edge Therapies

Gene therapy stands out as a beacon of hope in the fight against heart disease. Scientists are delving into ways to repair or replace faulty genes responsible for heart conditions, offering a glimpse of a future where permanent cures are within reach. Similarly, regenerative medicine holds promise in using stem cells to mend damaged heart tissue, potentially reversing the aftermath of heart attacks and failure.

Less Invasive Procedures, Greater Impact

The trend towards minimally invasive procedures continues to gather momentum. Techniques like transcatheter aortic valve replacement (TAVR) allow for valve repair or replacement without the need for open-heart surgery. These procedures mean shorter recovery times, reduced risks, and expanded access to treatment for patients previously deemed too high-risk for conventional surgery.

The Era of Personalized Medicine

Personalized medicine is transforming cardiac care. By analyzing a patient's genetic profile, lifestyle, and environment, doctors can tailor treatments to suit individual needs. This not only boosts treatment effectiveness but also minimizes side effects, enhancing overall quality of life.

Empowering Patients with Wearable Tech

Advances in wearable technology and remote monitoring are putting patients in the driver's seat of their heart health. Devices that track heart rhythm, blood pressure, and other vital signs provide real-time data for adjusting treatment plans as needed.

Harnessing AI and Machine Learning

Artificial intelligence (AI) and machine learning are revolutionizing cardiac diagnostics and treatment. AI algorithms analyze vast datasets to spot patterns and predict outcomes, leading to swifter interventions and more precise treatment strategies. Machine learning is even shaping personalized cardiac rehab programs that adapt to each patient's progress.

The Human Touch in Innovation

While technology takes center stage, it's the human element that truly drives these innovations. The dedication of researchers, the empathy of healthcare providers, and the resilience of patients are the heartbeats behind these advancements. It's the stories of recovery and perseverance that truly define the success of these breakthroughs.

Looking Ahead

The future of cardiac treatment holds boundless possibilities. With each leap in innovation, we draw closer to a world where heart disease is no longer a leading cause of mortality but a condition that can be effectively managed or even cured. While challenges lie ahead, the potential to save and enhance lives has never been greater.

CHAPTER ELEVEN

PREVENTING HEART DISEASE

11.1 Strategies for All Ages

Preventing heart disease is a lifelong journey that starts early and extends through all stages of life. It's about instilling habits that promote wellness and longevity, ensuring that heart health remains a priority for individuals of all ages. This chapter explores tailored strategies for each phase of life, aiming to make heart health accessible and achievable for everyone.

Early Childhood and Adolescence

The groundwork for heart health begins in childhood. Encouraging kids and teens to embrace healthy eating habits, stay active, and steer clear of sedentary habits sets the stage for a lifetime of wellness. Schools and parents can make a significant impact by providing nutritious meals and ample opportunities for physical activity. Educating young people about the dangers of smoking and substance abuse is also crucial during these formative years.

Young Adults

As individuals transition into adulthood, the choices they make profoundly influence their heart health in the long run. Young adults should prioritize regular exercise, a balanced diet, and stress management techniques as they navigate the demands of work and family life. Routine health screenings help identify risk factors like high blood pressure or cholesterol early on, allowing for timely intervention if needed.

Midlife Strategies

Midlife brings with it an increased risk of heart disease, making prevention efforts all the more crucial. More comprehensive health screenings and medical interventions, such as statins to manage cholesterol levels, may be necessary. Sustaining a healthy weight, managing stress effectively, and staying physically active are pivotal components of heart health during these years.

Senior Years

For seniors, preventing heart disease involves managing existing conditions while adjusting lifestyle habits to accommodate changes in physical abilities. Activities like walking, swimming, or tai chi can help maintain cardiovascular fitness, while dietary adjustments may be needed to meet changing nutritional needs. Social connections and community involvement play a significant role in fostering heart health and overall well-being.

Strategies Across All Ages

Certain strategies hold true regardless of age:

- No Smoking: Quitting smoking is one of the most impactful steps individuals can take to prevent heart disease.

- Healthy Diet: A diet rich in fruits, vegetables, lean proteins, and whole grains promotes heart health at any age.

- Regular Exercise: Engaging in physical activity, whether it's playing sports or going for walks, is essential for heart health.

- Stress Management: Developing healthy coping mechanisms for stress is key to maintaining heart health.

- Routine Check-Ups: Regular medical check-ups help identify and address risk factors before they escalate.

Community and Policy Initiatives

On a broader scale, community and policy initiatives are critical in promoting heart health. Public health campaigns that advocate for smoking cessation, access to nutritious foods, and opportunities for physical activity make a significant impact. Policies that regulate trans fats, curb tobacco use, and ensure healthcare access contribute to a healthier society overall.

Preventing heart disease is a collective effort that requires commitment from individuals and support from communities and policymakers alike. By adopting heart-healthy habits at every stage of life, we can reduce the prevalence of heart disease and create a healthier future for generations to come.

This chapter point to echo with readers of all ages, offering practical guidance and heartfelt encouragement. It's a call to action, urging everyone to prioritize heart health and support each other on this vital journey.

11.2 Community and Policy Initiatives

In the battle against heart disease, individual efforts matter, but the collective impact of community and policy initiatives is unparalleled. These broader strategies shape environments that support heart health and make healthy choices accessible to all.

The Strength of Community

Communities are the heartbeat of society, and their united efforts can yield remarkable results. Local projects like community gardens, farmers' markets, and public parks promote healthy lifestyles. Initiatives such as "walking school buses" not only encourage physical activity but also foster strong community bonds.

Policy: Molding Health Landscapes

Policies wield considerable influence on public health. Laws mandating clear nutritional labeling aid informed choices. Taxes on sugary drinks steer consumers towards healthier options. Smoke-free regulations safeguard non-smokers and incentivize smoking cessation.

Workplace Wellness Programs

Employers can significantly impact heart health through wellness programs. These initiatives offer health screenings, gym memberships, and smoking cessation support. By fostering a culture of health, workplaces promote healthy eating and physical activity.

Education and Awareness Campaigns

Education is pivotal in preventing heart disease. Culturally tailored campaigns, delivered through trusted channels, raise awareness about heart health risks and prevention strategies, motivating individuals to take proactive steps.

Advocacy and Healthcare Access

Advocacy groups ensure equitable access to healthcare. By advocating for improved policies and services, they break down barriers to care, ensuring that heart health remains a priority for policymakers.

Fostering Healthy Environments

Creating environments conducive to heart health is crucial. This involves designing cities with green spaces and safe biking lanes, offering nutritious food in schools, and ensuring communities have access to affordable healthy options.

The Role of Technology

Technology complements community and policy efforts. Mobile apps track physical activity, while social media campaigns disseminate heart-healthy messages, amplifying impact on a large scale.

Community and policy initiatives are linchpins in the fight against heart disease. Through collective action, we can cultivate a society that not only values heart health but also equips individuals with the resources needed for a heart-healthy life.

This chapter aims to inspire action, illustrating the myriad ways communities and policies collaborate to prevent heart disease. It underscores the importance of collective effort, reminding us that together, we can make a profound difference in heart health.

11.3 The Power of Prevention Education

Education stands as the bedrock of disease prevention, and in the realm of heart health, the impact of prevention education is profound. It's through education that individuals grasp the significance of lifestyle choices, the merits of early detection, and the steps they can take to diminish their risk of heart disease.

Grasping Heart Disease

Prevention education commences with unraveling the intricacies of heart disease and its physiological impact. It involves demystifying the condition, elucidating the role of arteries, the heart's function, and the consequences of malfunctions. Equipped with this foundational knowledge, individuals comprehend the weight of their daily decisions.

Lifestyle Choices: The Power to Shape Health

A pivotal facet of prevention education centers on lifestyle choices. It entails imparting awareness regarding the effects of diet, exercise, smoking, and alcohol on heart health. Educational endeavors often integrate practical demonstrations, such as contrasting healthy and unhealthy meal options or showcasing the effects of physical activity on heart rate.

Early Detection: The Importance of Vigilance

Education also champions early detection and screening initiatives. People need to be informed about available screenings, such as blood pressure checks and cholesterol tests, and understand the significance of initiating them at appropriate intervals. Recognizing the warning signs of heart disease and the value of routine check-ups are paramount.

Tailoring Education to Diverse Communities

Prevention education must be tailored to cater to diverse populations. Cultural sensitivity and linguistic accessibility are pivotal in ensuring that messages resonate across different communities. Programs should address the specific needs and apprehensions of varied groups, considering cultural dietary norms and traditional health perspectives.

Educational Endeavors in Schools

Educational institutions serve as fertile ground for prevention education. Integrating heart health into the curriculum can instill healthy habits early on. Initiatives like health fairs, culinary classes, and athletic activities render learning about heart health enjoyable and engaging for youngsters.

Promoting Heart Health in the Workplace

Workplaces emerge as another pivotal arena for prevention education. Employers can arrange seminars and workshops on heart health, furnish resources for stress management, and cultivate an environment conducive to a healthy lifestyle.

Community Outreach: Bringing Education to the Masses

Community outreach programs extend prevention education to broader demographics. These initiatives encompass complimentary screenings, health talks by medical experts, and collaborations with local establishments to endorse heart-healthy products and services.

Leveraging Digital Platforms for Education

In today's digital landscape, prevention education transcends physical boundaries. Websites, social media platforms, and mobile applications cater to a vast audience, offering interactive tools and resources to educate individuals about heart disease prevention.

The potency of prevention education lies in its capacity to drive behavioral change and preserve lives. It's not merely about imparting knowledge; it's about instigating action. Through investments in education, individuals can seize control of their heart health, paving the path towards a future where heart disease ceases to be a leading cause of mortality.

This chapter endeavors to resound with readers on a personal level, furnishing comprehensive insights into prevention education while underscoring its pivotal role in combatting heart disease. It's crafted to be both enlightening and motivational, urging readers to become champions for their own well-being and that of their communities.

CHAPTER TWELVE

THE FUTURE OF HEART HEALTH

12.1 Emerging Research and Theories

As we teeter on the brink of groundbreaking revelations, the future of heart health is unfolding through cutting-edge research and pioneering theories that challenge existing paradigms and usher in unprecedented possibilities. This chapter embarks on a journey through the frontiers of cardiac science, where innovation and inquiry promise to redefine our approach to preventing, diagnosing, and treating heart disease.

The Pursuit of Knowledge

At the heart of this endeavor lies the quest to decipher the intricacies of the cardiovascular system. Researchers delve into the molecular and genetic underpinnings of heart disease, striving to pinpoint biomarkers capable of predicting risk with unprecedented precision.

Unraveling Genetic Mysteries

Genetics emerges as a reservoir of invaluable insights. Scientists uncover how specific genetic variations influence susceptibility to heart conditions, aiming not only to identify risks but also to develop genetic therapies capable of preempting disease manifestation.

The Microbiome's Influence

Intriguingly, attention turns to the microbiome—a bustling ecosystem of microorganisms residing within us. Investigations unveil correlations between the gut microbiome's health and cardiac well-being, hinting at probiotic interventions poised to revolutionize heart health management.

Harnessing Artificial Intelligence

Artificial intelligence (AI) takes center stage in cardiology, with algorithms wielding unparalleled speed and accuracy in analyzing medical data and images. These

AI-powered tools empower clinicians to expedite diagnoses, ultimately enhancing patient outcomes.

Wearable Tech and Data Analytics

The ascent of wearable technology converges with big data analytics, heralding a new era in heart health surveillance. Through the aggregation and scrutiny of vast datasets from myriad users, researchers uncover latent patterns and insights, paving the way for tailored and proactive heart care strategies.

Lifestyle's Impact on Heart Health

Emerging studies underscore lifestyle's pivotal role in heart health. Investigations explore how factors like sleep, stress, and social connections influence cardiac well-being, fostering a holistic approach to disease prevention that transcends mere symptomatic management.

Innovative Treatment Modalities

On the treatment front, technological advancements redefine therapeutic landscapes. From 3D-printed cardiac valves to nanotechnology-enabled targeted drug delivery, the horizon brims with possibilities poised to revolutionize heart disease management.

Boundary-Pushing Theories

Theoretical explorations push the envelope of conventional wisdom. Some researchers contemplate heart disease as an autoimmune ailment, while others delve into the regenerative potential of stem cells in healing cardiac tissue.

The Human Element

Amidst this scientific odyssey, the human narrative remains paramount. It's the tales of patients, the dedication of healthcare practitioners, and the tenacity of researchers that propel this pursuit forward. Each breakthrough epitomizes the transformative impact of research and innovation on human lives.

In Closing

The future of heart health gleams with the promise of burgeoning research and visionary theories. As we traverse the frontiers of cardiovascular science, we edge closer to a realm where heart disease transcends its status as a leading cause of mortality, poised to be conquered through enlightenment, empathy, and relentless exploration.

12.2 The Evolution of Heart Care

The evolution of heart care is a testament to human innovation and compassion, a saga spanning centuries from ancient wisdom to modern marvels. Join us on this journey through the milestones of cardiac care, where breakthroughs have rewritten the narrative of heart disease and transformed countless lives.

Early Explorations

Our tale begins with the ancients, who revered the heart's significance while grappling with its mysteries. It wasn't until luminaries like William Harvey in the Renaissance era that we began to decipher the secrets of circulation. Despite this, treatments remained rudimentary, often limited to rest and folk remedies.

The Dawn of Modern Cardiology

The 20th century ushered in the dawn of modern cardiology. The invention of the electrocardiogram (ECG) by Willem Einthoven provided a pivotal tool for understanding cardiac function. Pioneers like Dr. John Gibbon performed groundbreaking open-heart surgeries, setting the stage for a new era of cardiac interventions.

Interventional Innovations

The latter half of the 20th century witnessed the rise of interventional cardiology. Innovations like angioplasty, pioneered by Dr. Andreas Gruentzig, offered less invasive alternatives to traditional surgery. The advent of coronary stents further propelled this progress, transforming the landscape of cardiovascular care.

Embracing Prevention

With growing insights into heart disease, prevention emerged as a cornerstone of cardiac care. Landmark studies like the Framingham Heart Study unveiled key risk factors, sparking public health initiatives worldwide. Through education and advocacy, countless lives have been safeguarded against the ravages of cardiovascular illness.

Medicinal Milestones

Pharmaceutical breakthroughs have also left an indelible mark on heart care. From the discovery of statins to the development of blood thinners and beta-blockers, medications have become indispensable allies in managing heart conditions, offering hope and longevity to patients worldwide.

The Digital Renaissance

Enter the digital age, heralding a new frontier in heart care. Wearable devices provide real-time insights into heart health, while telemedicine bridges the gap between patients and providers. Artificial intelligence lends its prowess to diagnostics and treatment, heralding a future of personalized medicine.

Heartfelt Heroes

Amidst the scientific strides, it's the human element that resonates most deeply—the resilience of patients, the dedication of healthcare professionals, and the compassion that binds them together. Their stories echo through the annals of cardiac history, driving progress and inspiring hope.

A Glimpse of Tomorrow

Peering into the future, we glimpse a horizon ripe with promise. Gene editing, regenerative therapies, and nanotechnology hold the keys to unlocking a world where heart disease is no longer a scourge but a conquerable foe. The evolution of heart care is an ever-unfolding saga, fueled by our relentless pursuit of healing and understanding.

In Closing

The evolution of heart care is a testament to human resilience and determination. It's a testament to our unwavering commitment to rewriting the story of heart disease—one of progress, hope, and the enduring spirit of humanity. As we stand on the threshold of tomorrow, let us carry forward the torch of discovery, illuminating the path to a future where every heartbeat is a testament to life's triumphs.

This chapter is penned to resonate with readers on a personal level, intertwining the technical advancements of heart care with the poignant narratives that breathe life into the science. It's a tribute to the past, a celebration of the present, and a beacon of hope for the future, all narrated through the lens of our shared humanity.

12.3 A Vision for a Heart-Healthy Society

Imagine a world where every heartbeat resonates with vitality, where the rhythm of life pulses with the promise of well-being. This chapter invites you to envision a future where heart health isn't just a goal but a reality—a world where society's heartbeat echoes the harmony of health and happiness.

At the core of this vision lies education and awareness—a society where knowledge empowers individuals to make heart-smart choices. From farm to table, from playground to workplace, every facet of life nurtures cardiovascular wellness, fostering a culture where hearts thrive.

Nourishing Nutrition

In this imagined future, nutrition reigns supreme. Food systems prioritize wholesome, nourishing fare, making heart-healthy options accessible to all. Supermarkets brim with fresh produce, while culinary education programs instill the art of heart-healthy cooking, enriching communities with the joy of shared meals.

Embracing Active Living

Physical activity isn't just a habit; it's a way of life. Cities are designed for movement, with green spaces and bike lanes inviting daily exercise. Workplaces champion active breaks, and technological innovations make fitness fun and inclusive, ensuring that every step is a stride toward heart health.

Accessible, Personalized Healthcare

Healthcare evolves into a proactive, personalized partnership. Preventive screenings become routine, and telemedicine erases geographic barriers, extending care to every corner. With a focus on individual needs and genetic insights, treatment becomes tailored, ensuring that every heartbeat receives the attention it deserves.

Mental Wellness: Nurturing the Heart-Mind Connection

Mental well-being takes center stage, recognized as integral to heart health. Stress management and emotional support are woven into healthcare, fostering balance and resilience. Societies prioritize holistic well-being, acknowledging the profound interplay between mind and heart.

Community: The Heartbeat of Unity

Communities pulse with vitality, nurturing connections that sustain the soul. Initiatives promote social cohesion, fostering support networks that uplift every member. Guided by policies that prioritize health and harmony, societies flourish as collective stewards of heart health.

Global Solidarity: Uniting Against Heart Disease

This vision transcends borders, uniting nations in the fight against heart disease. Through shared knowledge and collaborative action, countries pool resources to tackle cardiovascular challenges. International policies address social determinants, striving to dismantle barriers to heart health worldwide.

A heart-healthy society isn't a distant dream; it's within our grasp. It calls for collective action, fueled by passion and purpose. As we gaze into the future, let us carry this vision—a vision of a world where every heartbeat pulses with vitality, where health is cherished as society's most precious treasure.

This chapter is penned to inspire and ignite, kindling the flames of hope for a heart-healthy tomorrow. It beckons each of us to become architects of this vision, forging a future where every beat is a symphony of well-being and every heart sings with the joy of vitality.

CONCLUSION

As we draw the curtains on this enlightening voyage through the realms of heart health, we stand in awe of the extraordinary strides and infinite possibilities that stretch out in the field of cardiology. From the humble beginnings of basic comprehension to the dazzling advancements of the present day, we have been privileged witnesses to the remarkable transformation of cardiac care.

Reflecting upon the narratives woven throughout this book, both from a scientific lens and through the prism of personal experience, it becomes abundantly clear that the essence of heart health transcends the boundaries of medical science; it is, at its core, a profoundly human pursuit. We've journeyed through the influence of daily lifestyle choices on heart disease, immersed ourselves in the significance of community engagement and policy reforms in prevention, and cast our gaze towards a prospect where each heartbeat resonates with the fullness of life.

Visualize a parent, who, equipped with the insights gleaned from these pages, revolutionizes their family's nutritional habits, trading in the convenience of processed foods for the nourishment of natural, home-cooked meals, and finds joy in the simple act of walking through the local park. Consider a farmer in a remote village, who, through the wonders of telemedicine, gains access to critical cardiac care, a blessing once deemed beyond reach. Contemplate a young student, whose education in heart health ignites a lifelong passion, shaping them into a champion for community wellness.

These vignettes of everyday life capture the profound resonance of knowledge, empathy, and innovation in the sphere of heart care. As we cast our eyes towards the path ahead, let us hold tight to the wisdom imparted within these chapters—a pledge to lifelong learning, a commitment to nurturing our communities, and an unceasing quest for a world where every pulsation is a celebration of health and contentment.

The future of heart health rests in our collective hands, beckoning us to author the forthcoming narrative in this epic tale of advancement and optimism. With hearts wide open and resolve unshaken, let us unite in this noble endeavor, confident in the knowledge that together, we possess the capacity to forge a society where the cadence of existence harmonizes with the melody of heart-centered living.

"Thanks for reading! If you enjoyed this book or found it useful, I'd be very grateful if you'd post a short review on Amazon. Your support really does make a difference and I read all the reviews personally so I can get your feedback and make this book even better.